LifeEnergy Recipes

Blending Your Way to Optimum Health

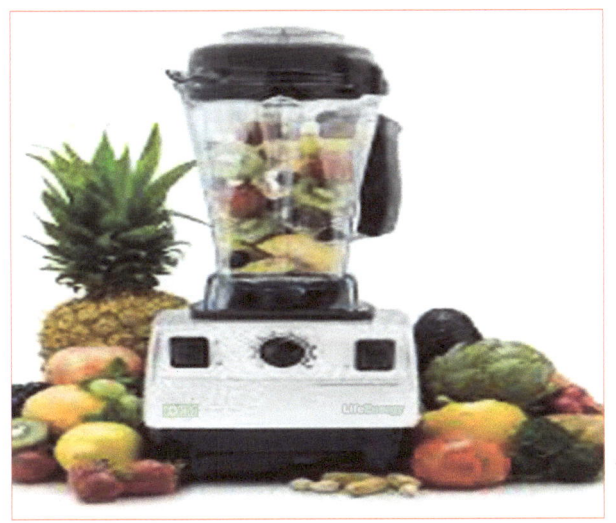

lifestyle of health and sustainability

Super-Easy ♥ *Super-Delicious* ♥ *Low Calorie*
Super-Nutritious Blended Drinks

~

Yvonne Tolstoy

LifeEnergy Recipes

Blending Your Way to Optimum Health

Yvonne Tolstoy

IAM PUBLISHING

USA

Printed in the United States of America
First Printing: 2014
ISBN-13: 978-1502407993

IAM Publishing
USA

www.LifeEnergyUSA.com
Photos by: Randy Mayor

Contents

To Blend or Not to Blend...

that is the Question!

Introduction

Why Blend? Using the LifeEnergy blender has many benefits: it saves time, it's fast, easy and convenient; think of it as "fast food" that is very nutritious and delicious. Individuals, both young and mature, can quickly boost their daily intake of vital nutrients using the LifeEnergy Blender. Depending on your health objective, whether you are wanting to supplement your diet, detox, do a cleansing fast, drop some extra pounds, stop disease or reverse aging - blending is a quick, easy and fun way to do it.

Blending foods is not only fun, it is an easy way to increase life-energy, and improve your overall well-being. Using the LifeEnergy blender assists the body in building strong cellular structures, healthy organs, glands and body systems. Blending foods increases the nutritional content of your beverages; you will experience more energy, and feel more alert, while supporting healthy immune function and digestion. Many people report numerous health benefits, including improvements in their eyesight, hair, skin, and nails. It can help reduce stress, promote sleep, and improve fitness recovery.

Blending your foods increases vitamin, enzyme, protein and mineral intake, and puts you on the fast-track to achieving optimum health. When blending fruits, vegetables, sprouts, grains, nuts or seeds you increase the nutrient content of your beverages. Blended beverages are very nutrient dense, having a concentration of all the necessary elements needed to build a strong, lean, healthy body. It's also a great way to get our children to drink their fruits and vegetables - and like it! Using the LifeEnergy Blender is also ideal for making healthy "baby foods."

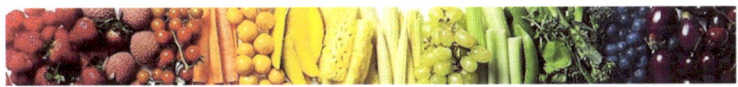

So the question is no longer "to blend or not to blend" but rather…

…are you ready to get started?

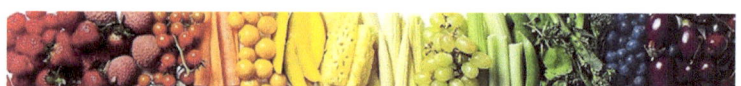

Chapter 1

Getting Started
Before Using Your LifeEnergy Blender

Not all blenders are created equal. With the LifeEnergy Blender you can make soups, nut butters, nut milks, smoothies, creams, green drinks, dressings, frozen desserts, batters, breads, and even flour. Use the LE Blender to warm foods, blend, chop, churn, cream, crush, grind, mix, puree, and whip when creating your favorite recipes

R-E-S-P-E-C-T
Although the LifeEnergy Blender is powerful enough to effectively blend the toughest of ingredients, soaking your ingredients and cutting up your vegetables will prevent undue stress, and ensure maximum durability and longevity - treat it with respect and it will serve you for a long time. Whether your whirling up your favorite smoothie or pulverizing nuts, it will go much better if you properly prepare the ingredients.

Layering
Layering ingredients makes for efficient blending. Always put liquids in first, followed by powders and soft ingredients, and last but not least the hardest ingredients on top. Liquids first, allows the blades to quickly work when you first turn on the blender. Follow with powdered ingredients, so upon ignition they don't fly up and get stuck to the blender's lid. Then add your soft foods like fruits, and leafy greens, and finally add your hard ingredients like raw veggies, frozen fruits, and ice. Adding ice last prevents over-blending, and keeps the consistency from becoming too watery.

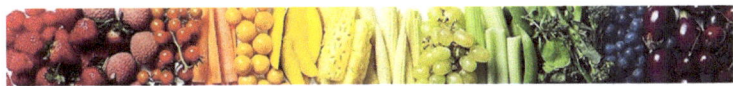

1

Layering allows the blades to pull all the ingredients together for a perfect blend. Keep in mind as you layer it on, not to over-fill the container, or under-fill it. Too much and the contents will not have the room needed to blend, and with too little content the blades will not be immersed, and will just spin with no effect.

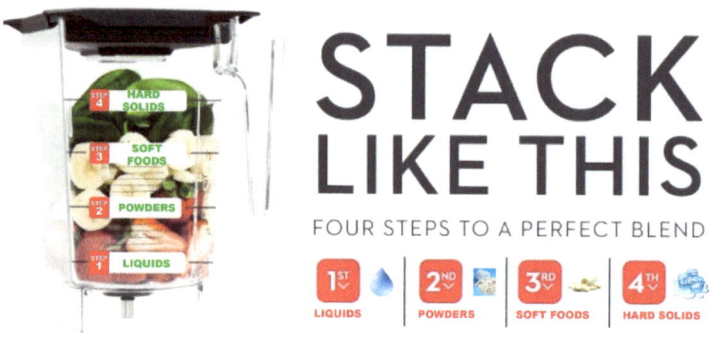

Prep & Soak

When it comes to preparing your fruits and veggies, very little preparation is necessary when using the LifeEnergy Blender due to its powerful motor. Of course you want to wash your produce, but most produce can be added whole, with the exception of your larger produce like pineapple.

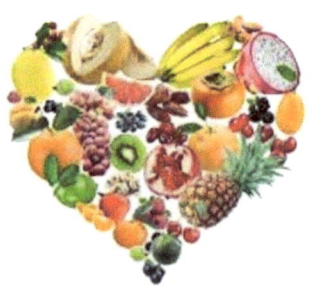

DO NOT put peach or cherry pits in your blender; however, avocado, apples, and citrus can go in whole, with seeds

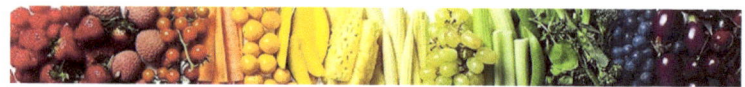

and pits included. While there is some controversy regarding the cyanogen found in apple seeds, scientific studies have shown that over 30 native herbs from around the world contain cyanogens, which are noted for having anti-cancer properties. Another good reason to use the whole fruit is that many of the important nutrients are found in the skin, core, and other parts typically discarded. Although many may object to this suggestion with extreme verbosity, I'm going to continue blending my whole fruits and veggies to maximize the health benefits - I highly recommend it.

Soaking nuts, seeds, grains, dehydrated foods, dried fruit, dates and other fibrous foods over-night is always a good idea. Soaking these food items will also enhance the texture and enzymatic activity of your foods. Soaked dates and sun-dried tomatoes blend more easily and deliver more flavor.

Soaking raw nuts and seeds increases the nutritional content of Vitamins A, B, & C. When soaking almonds, cashews, macadamia, and other nuts it offers a wonderful creamy texture, but also makes the final product more digestible by activating enzymatic function, and removing toxic inhibitors inherent within the nuts.

Soaking Chart		
Almond	12	Hours
Brazil Nuts	2	Hours
Cashews	2	Hours
Chia Seeds	2	Hours
Flax Seeds	2	Hours
Hazel Nuts	8	Hours
Hemp Seeds	0	Hours
Macadamia Nuts	2	Hours
Pecans	8	Hours
Pine Nuts	2	Hours
Pistachios	4	Hours
Pumpkin Seeds	6	Hours
Sesame Seeds	6	Hours
Sunflower Seeds	4	Hours
Walnuts	8	Hours
Wild Jungle Peanuts	8	Hours

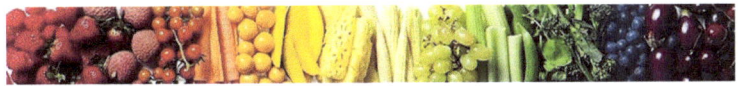

It's also very beneficial to add a little salt to the water you will be using for soaking. Soaking nuts and seeds in warm salted water activates beneficial enzymes, while neutralizing the enzyme inhibitors making them more digestible.

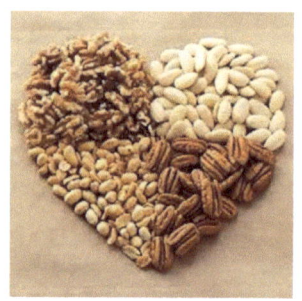

Soaking grains in pure water with a little lemon juice or apple cider vinegar diluted in water also encourages the production of enzymes, which neutralizes phytic acids that strain the digestive system.

While soaking, keep the nuts, grains or seeds in the dark, and at room temperature. It is a good idea to keep the container in which you are soaking the nuts or seeds covered. Using a jar with a lid is ideal, or if using a bowl place a towel, or plate over it.

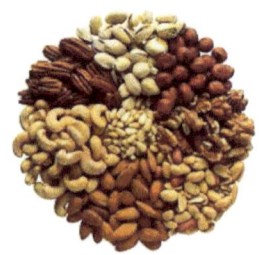

After soaking, pour off the water, and rinse the nuts and seeds very well. Rinse soaked nuts or seeds in a colander, and place under running water, continue until the water draining from the colander is clear. A final rinse with apple cider vinegar is recommended to remove any bacteria.

As a rule, soaking nuts and seeds for 8-12 hours is ideal; however, softer nuts and seeds require less soaking time. Place desired amount of nuts or seeds in a bowl or jar, and cover with room temperature distilled, purified or filtered water. Add a teaspoon of Himalayan or Celtic Sea Salt to the water. A good ratio would be 2:1, two parts water to 1 part nuts.

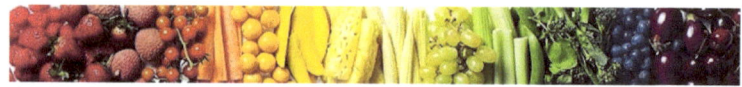

It's also important to soak dried fruit before blending, only because it is very hard for the body to digest and assimilate dried foods that are dehydrated. Soaking dried fruit over-night before using is always a good idea. If the dried fruit is not rehydrated, your body will give up fluids to rehydrate the food during digestion, this can cause dehydration. Fresh fruit is always the best choice, but if you choose dried fruit be sure to soak, and buy only organic to avoid toxic oils and additives.

Keep it Raw

Raw nuts contain essential fats that contribute to healthy arteries and brain function. When roasted, heated or pasteurized these fats become free radicals contributing to arterial plaque and cardiovascular disease. So when it comes to your nuts - keep it raw!

Some Like it Hot

Having said all that, when working with hot soups or sauces it is a good idea to blend in batches, not over-filling the blender. This reduces the risk of being scalded, saves time, and keeps it neat.

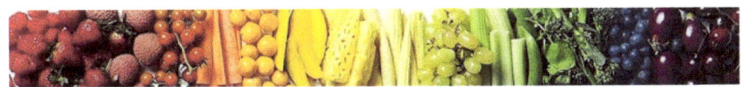

Chapter 2

Blending the Rainbow
Colors Count

When choosing foods, select foods with a variety of colors. When choosing ingredients for your smoothie it is best to use fresh, organic produce. If fresh is not available then frozen is the next best thing.

Many individuals like their smoothies cold, rather than using ice, adding frozen fruits to your smoothie is a great alternative. I never recommend using canned goods.

Nature has provided a full spectrum of colorful foods, rich in health-promoting nutrients. Most fresh fruits need not be peeled, like apples, pears, grapes, kiwi and whole berries, watermelon, and yes even pineapple.

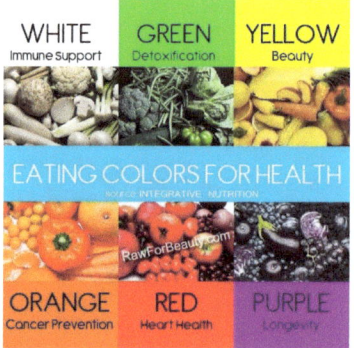

Whereas for other fruits like citrus, it is a good idea to leave as much of the pith (white covering under the outer peel) on - many of the essential nutrients are just below the outer peel. Using package frozen fruit is also an option, but fresh, organic is always preferred.

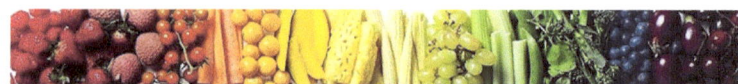

6

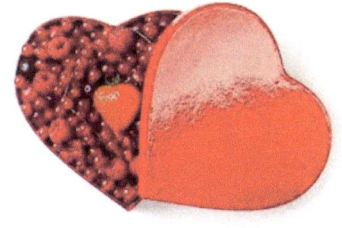

Red fruits and vegetables get their color from something called flavanoids: lycopene and anythocyanins, which have powerful cancer-fighting and antioxidant properties. Red produce is most notable for it's high levels of vitamin A, vitamin C, Manganese, and Fiber. Red fruits and vegetables improves memory, lung function, joints, and lowers LDL cholesterol, blood pressure, and free radicals.

Orange and **Yellow** fruits and vegetables contain beta-carotene (a form of vitamin A). Orange and yellow fruits and

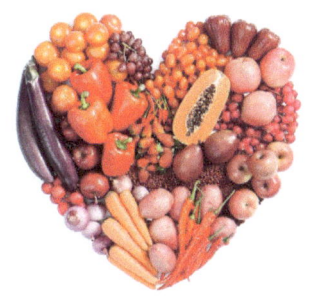

vegetables are also colored with carotenoids. This group is high in Vitamin A and C, just like their red buddies. They also are typically abundant in fiber, significant levels of manganese, potassium, and various B vitamins.

Yellow produce contains more vitamin C and less vitamin A than orange produce. Orange and yellow produce is great for our immune system, heart health, vision, skin health, and has age reversing properties. Orange and yellow produce also helps lower LDL cholesterol, blood pressure, and free radicals.

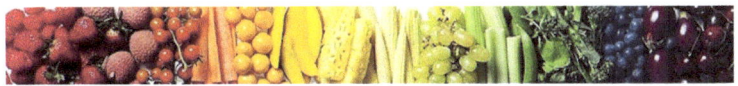

Tan, white and colorless produce gets its pigment from anthoxanthin, beta-glucans, lignans and other chemical compounds. Though void of color, these foods are not void of nutrients. In fact, these fruits and vegetables provide tremendous immune support, as they are filled with anti-bacterial, anti-fungal, and anti-viral properties. You'll also find vitamin C, vitamin K, folate, and fiber in this group.

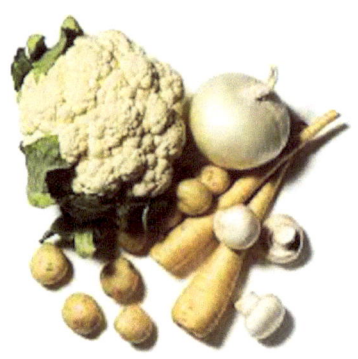

Although colorless, these fruits and vegetables have properties that reduce the risk of various cancers, balance hormone levels, and boost our immune system. These foods are packed with vitamin B6, choline, iron, magnesium, phosphorus, potassium and, sodium, and are high in protein.

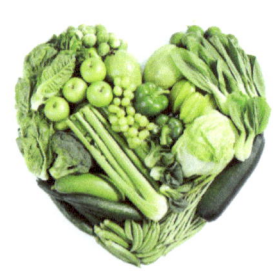

Green produce is probably the most celebrated of foods, due to their high content of chlorophyll, a powerful compound that is very similar to hemoglobin in molecular structure. Green foods fight cell damage, and is filled with vitamin K, vitamin C, numerous B vitamins, and just about every nutritional element, including, calcium, and potassium. Green produce, especially leafy greens, are full of fiber too.

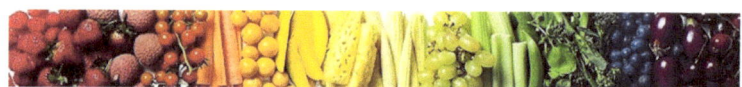

Green produce is great for aiding digestion, improving the immune system, and is most beneficial for our vision, bones, and teeth. Greens can lower your LDL cholesterol and blood pressure, and help fight diabetes, and promote heart health. High in vitamin B2, B3, B5, B6, and B9, as well as vitamin E, potassium, iron, magnesium, manganese, phosphorus, and zinc.

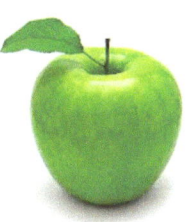

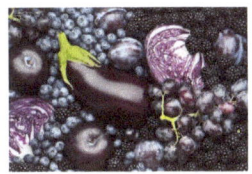

Blue and **Purple** produce comes from anthocyancins, which are powerful antioxidants. They also contain other phytochemincals and flavanoids such as lutein, zeaxanthin, resveratrol, ellagic acid, quercentin, and powerful antioxidants.

Blue and purple produce have tremendous cancer-fighting properties, considerable fiber, and high content of vitamin C, vitamin K, manganese, calcium, iron, magnesium, phosphorus, and potassium, as well as significant levels of vitamin E, and folic acid - just to name a few.

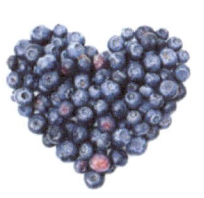

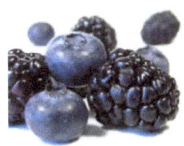

The blue group is great for improving memory, brain function, and fighting inflammation. **Blue** and **Purple** foods are reported to improve immune function, aide in digestion, reverse aging, and support heart health.

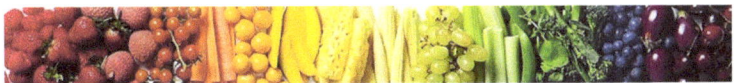

Eating a variety of colors is essential to a vibrant, healthy life. These foods are anti-carcinogenic, and can help slow, stop, or even reverse cancerous cell growth. Not only are the colors good for you, they are very pretty as well, and will make you pretty too - inside and out!

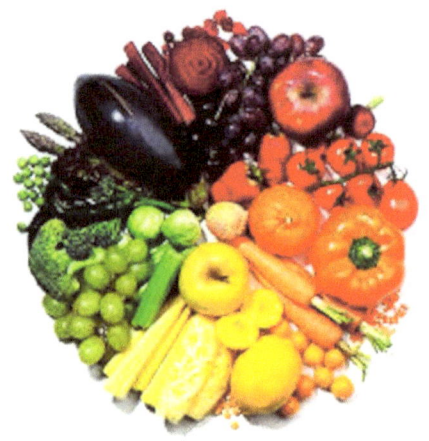

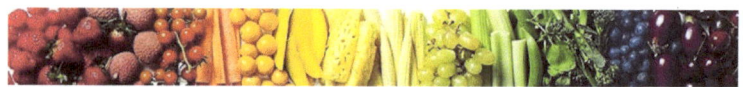

Chapter 3

Healthy Additions
Super Power Foods

What are Super-foods? Super foods are foods that make us feel SUPER-GOOD! Super-foods provide potent nutrients in unique combinations and quantities, promoting wellness, healthy body weight, and contain multiple disease-fighting nutrients, without excess calories. Super-foods are easy to incorporate into our diet. Eaten regularly, these foods will satisfy all the dietary recommendations of nutrients that are typically missing from our standard American diets (SAD).

Any number of super-foods may be added to your smoothie to boost its nutritional content. Some of my favorite additions include: bee pollen, cayenne, coconut, hemp, ginger, goji berries, maca, schisandra and turmeric. While some of these super foods are a bit exotic, most can be found on the website: www.PerfectHealthSolutions.us

Bee Pollen is a potent food, it is 40% protein, in the form of free amino acids that are readily available for use in the human body. It is considered one of nature's most complete foods, being that it contains all the essential components of life. 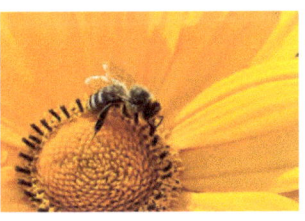 Bee pollen is remarkably rejuvenating, and has anti-cancer qualities, correcting nutritional deficiencies and imbalances. Science has yet to identify all of the nutritious elements present in pollen, but that is no reason to keep us from enjoying its many benefits.

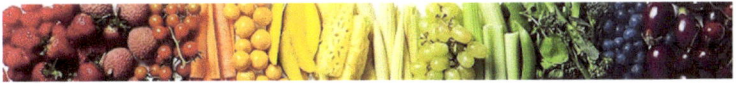

Cayenne is a spice for those who like it hot! Considered very therapeutic in the Americas and China, it contains many powerful compounds. Used for a variety of ailments including heartburn, delirium, tremors, gout, paralysis, fever, dyspepsia, coughs, sore

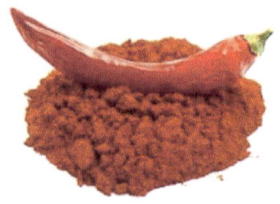

throats, flatulence, hemorrhoids, nausea, fever and ulcers. It has anti-fungal properties, anti-bacterial, and anti-irritant properties, and is known as a circulatory stimulant. It increases the pulse of lymphatic and digestive rhythms, thus very useful in detoxifying the body. Adding a pinch of cayenne to our smoothies can be particularly helpful in relieving joint pain, supporting weight loss and normalizing blood pressure, while promoting heart-health.

Coconut has many health benefits, it taste great, and provides an immediate source of energy with a low glycemic index. From the inside-out the unique properties of coconut reduces stress, cholesterol, and obesity. It boosts the immune system, supports proper digestion, and regulates metabolism. It also provides relief from kidney problems, heart diseases, high blood pressure, diabetes, HIV, and cancer, while helping to improve dental quality, and bone strength.

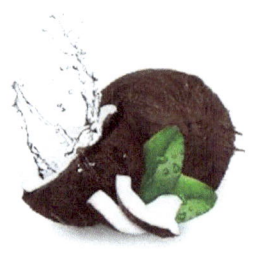

The benefits of coconut can be attributed to the presence of lauric acid, capric acid and caprylic acid, and its antimicrobial, antioxidant, anti-fungal, antibacterial, and soothing qualities.

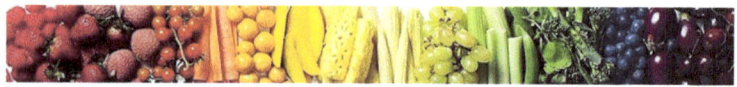

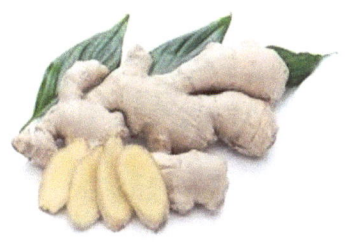

Ginger has a long history and tradition of being very effective as an herbal medicine. Regarded as a carminative and intestinal spasmolytic, it promotes elimination of intestinal gas and relaxes and soothes the intestinal lining.

Ginger possesses many therapeutic properties including anti-inflammatory, and antioxidant effects. Ginger has been known to reduce nausea, vomiting, motion sickness, indigestion, muscular discomfort, and inflammation, protecting against colorectal cancer.

Goji berries are very rich in nutrients, some consider it the fountain of youth. Used to treat many health issues like diabetes, high blood pressure, fever, athletic performance, mental health and age related eye disorders. Goji contains many nutrients and phytochemicals including eleven essential and twenty-two trace dietary minerals. Goji is very high in Vitamin C, calcium, potassium, iron, zinc, selenium, Vitamin B2, beta-carotene (Vitamin A), and 18 amino acids. Goji

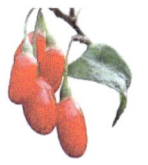

also contains antioxidants that may prevent the growth of cancer cells, reduce blood glucose, protect the liver, improve sexual function, boost immune function, promote weight loss, lower cholesterol and promote longevity. Some berries are very dry, thus soaking your berries is a good idea, using the soaked berries, and the water they are soaked in makes for a great addition to any smoothie.

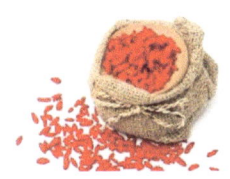

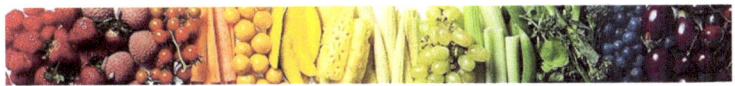

Hemp also has a long history of diverse uses, it has been consumed for centuries, and highly regarded for the many essential nutrients it possesses. Its reputation continues to flourish as its many health benefits continue to be revealed.

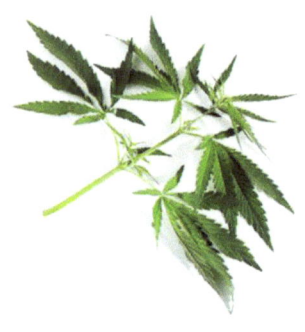

Hemp is considered a complete protein because it contains all eight essential amino acids. This makes it a good protein source for vegetarians and vegans. Hemp protein is easy to digest, unlike soy or whey, which contain inhibitors that block absorption, and can cause indigestion, intestinal toxemia, and allergic reactions in many people; whereas hemp has no known allergens and does not cause intestinal toxemia.

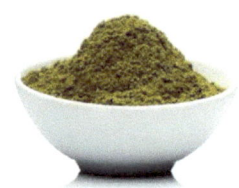

Hemp also contains vital vitamins, minerals, fibre, enzymes, probiotics, antioxidants and essential fatty acids (Omega-3 and Omega-6). It is a high-fiber protein, considered superior due to its above average digestibility. Hemp enhances immune potential and has anti-fatigue properties, and is very effective at improving kidney function.

Hemp is a nutrient dense food that supports a healthy, active lifestyle improving muscle control, mental function, and normal body maintenance of cells, tissues and organs.

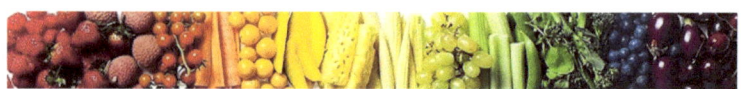

Maca is a root belonging to the radish family, and is very rich in Vitamin B, Vitamin C and Vitamin E. It provides generous amounts of calcium, zinc, iron, magnesium, phosphorous and amino acids. Widely used to promote hormonal balance, it serves to boost libido, increase endurance and fertility.

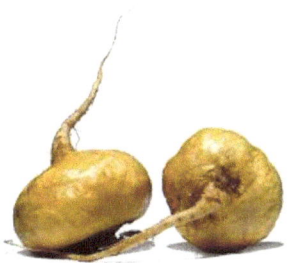

Maca has been used to relieve menstrual cramps, and menopausal symptoms of body pain, hot flashes, anxiety, mood swings and depression. When using maca, it should be introduced into the diet slowly. After several days of use energy levels may increase.

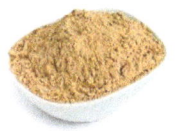

Known as Peruvian Ginseng, it has become the subject of much research. Overall health benefits may include reversing anemia, and cardiovascular diseases since maca restores red blood cells. It is reported to support bone health, and allows wounds to heal more quickly.

Maca is not recommended for pregnant or lactating women.

Schisandra is the ultimate berry, being revered as strong medicine in Russia, and used in China for over 2000 years. It is an exotic sweet, sour, salty, bitter and pungent fruit that has many medicinal properties. Schisandra has traditionally

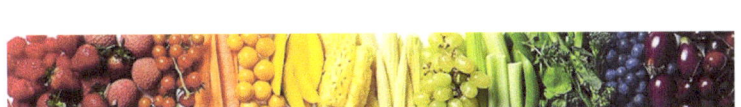

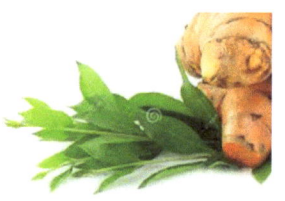

been used for longevity and vitality, it possesses antioxidant, anti-inflammatory, and adaptogenic properties. It helps maintain all the cells in the body, and is included in many herbal formulas to reduce stress, improve energy and support mental health. In various clinical studies it was demonstrated to have superior mind-sharpening powers.

Studies indicate schisandra is a potent tonic, decreasing fatigue and enhancing physical and mental performance, improving concentration and coordination. Schisandra is superior in protecting the liver. Used for millennia to retard the aging process, and as a sexual tonic, schisandra is indeed a true feel-good berry.

Turmeric is considered a spice, it has many beneficial properties. It is a natural anti-inflammatory, antibiotic, antiseptic, anti-arthritic, and analgesic. Often used to treat stomach disorders, arthritis and other inflammatory diseases.

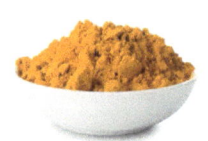

Studies in China conclude that consumption of turmeric helps lower cholesterol, improves blood flow, strengthens blood vessels, speeds wound healing, improves digestion, aids in fat metabolism and weight management.

Turmeric is also reported to reduce side effects of chemotherapy, and slows the progression of Multiple-sclerosis. It has many anti-cancer properties, and has been shown to

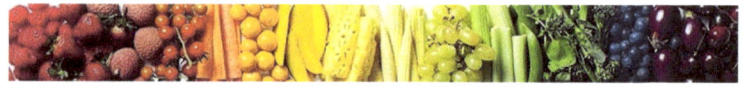

have a positive effect on Parkinson's and Alzheimer's disease, reducing amyloid plaque by as much as 50%.

Other super-foods, which can be used in our smoothies to promote, and sustain health, and longevity include:

• Acai	• Green Tea
• Alfalfa	• Honey
• Almonds	• Kale
• Ashwagandha	• Kiwi
• Avocado	• Lemon
• Barley Grass	• Lucuma
• Beets	• Maple Syrup
• Blueberries	• Mangosteen
• Broccoli	• Molasses
• Chia Seeds	• Noni
• Chlorella	• Pineapple
• Cinnamon	• Pomegranate
• Cranberries	• Raspberries
• Flax Seeds	• Strawberries
• Garlic	• Wheatgrass
• Greek Yogurt	• Quinoa

Some of you may be asking, why cacao (*aka: cocoa, chocolat, chocolate,*) did not make the cut as a super-food in this book? Reason being is that cacao is a TOXIN. Since 1979, I have spoken out

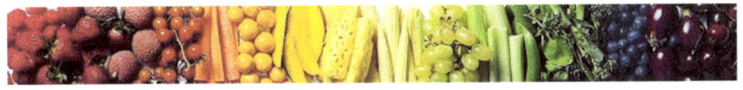

against cacao, while promoting the virtues of Carob. That is not to say that I don't enjoy the sweet, rich, creamy temptation of a good bitter chocolate from time to time; however, there is always a price to pay - it is not part of a healthy lifestyle.

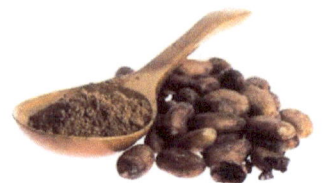

Many individuals may extol the nutrients present in cacao; however, there's no way around it, it is a drug - and a very stimulating one at that. It is systemically toxic, especially to the liver, kidneys and adrenals.

Cacao is a stimulant, it is one of the most addictive substances known. After consuming this highly processed substance, immediately the adrenals kick into high gear, releasing stress hormones to the point of exhausting the adrenals. In addition, cacao obstructs the kidneys, inhibiting normal function.

When cacao is consumed the liver literally cringes and shrivels; such responses occur as the body fights to quickly eliminate the toxic substance ingested. No matter how you cut it, eating chocolate, or "raw" cacao, on a regular basis is not healthy.

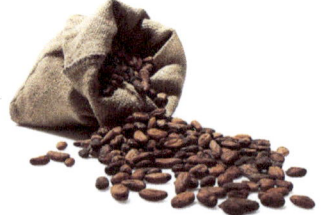

Although cacao has taken the raw food movement by storm it is anything but "raw", and more importantly it must not be considered as a food. It is a complex plant that must be highly processed, cooked and fermented

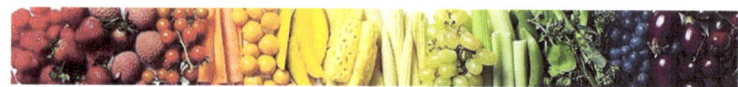

prior to consumption. A bean like seed, cacao initially was domesticated as a ceremonial, alcoholic beverage. Domestication of cacao originated in Peru; however, it was the pulp surrounding the cacao seed that was consumed after being cooked, and fermented to produce a mildly alcoholic, hallucinogenic beverage.

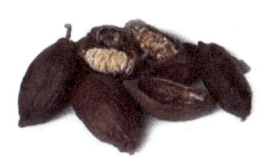

It was believed to be toxic for women and children and was only used by men in their sacrificial offerings to their gods. After drinking the intoxicating beverage, priests would lance their ear lobes and cover the cacao seed with their blood; rather than eat the seeds they offered it as a suitable sacrifice to their gods.

It's really a no-brainer! Instead of cacao, try carob. Cacao contains caffeine or theobromine, both of these chemicals (which belong to a family of substances called methylxanthines) are stimulants; while caffeine works primarily on the central nervous system, theobromine stimulates the cardiovascular and pulmonary systems. Many will argue that the stimulating effects of cacao are desired, yet this argument fails to justify the damaging effects of cacao, which far outweigh cacao's limited perceived benefits.

Years ago, I had a discussion with Brian Clement of the Hippocrates Health Institute regarding cacao. At the time he was a big promoter of "raw" cacao. Clement was one of many who advocated cacao, and championed it's publicity. During a presentation, where Clement was extolling the benefits of cacao, I publicly opposed his protagonist views of cacao, and presented the case against it; I was ridiculed, scoffed and shunned.

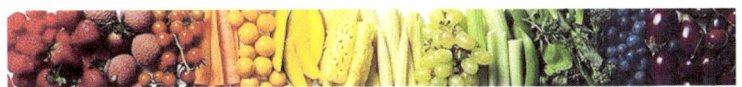

Years after the fact, Mr. Clement has changed his tune, and now speaks out against cacao - all I can say is "better late than never" - he now joins many others considered to be "authorities" in their field, teaching the truth about the toxic effects of cacao, which for years was rejected, and still is by many in the raw food circles. My advice to you: Make Truth Your Authority - Not Authorities Your Truth!

Proponents of "raw" cacao claim there is a difference between "raw" and refined chocolate, stating raw cacao contains high levels of antioxidants and minerals, while refined chocolate does not. Regardless of whether we are talking about refined chocolate, dark chocolate or "raw" cacao the facts remain conclusive - the overall nutritional value of a food determines its level of healthiness, not just a few components.

The negative aspects inherent in cacao, in any form, far outweigh the positive. Thus when considering whether to include cacao as a super-food, think again. For a substance to be a super-food it must first "do no harm", and it must have an abundance of nutrients. If the toxins outweigh the nutrients then we can not classify it as a super-food.

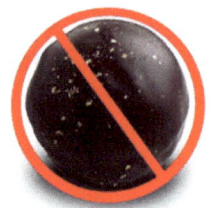

Still not convinced, a simple pH test of the urine and saliva, 24 hours after eating chocolate or cacao may be indicative enough to change your mind. I challenge you to take the cacao pH test and see for yourself - I think you'll be surprised to find the pH swings acid every time. In addition, when cacao is consumed the count of white blood cells triple, an indicator that the body considers it a foreign

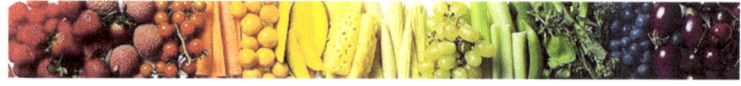

invader, a toxin that must be neutralized. This fact alone, makes the case *against* cacao as a super-food - case closed!

As you continue to explore the many TRUE super-foods, I'm sure you too will have your favorites. I encourage you however, stick to the real super-foods: leafy greens, fruits, veggies, herbs and spices.

Super Foods. . .

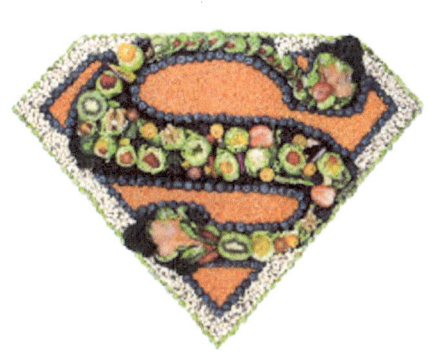

Will make you feel S-U-P-E-R!!

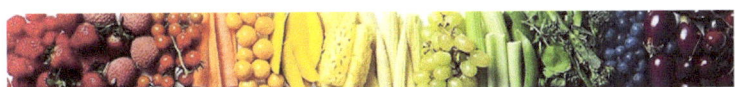

Chapter 4

Go Green
Super Green Smoothies

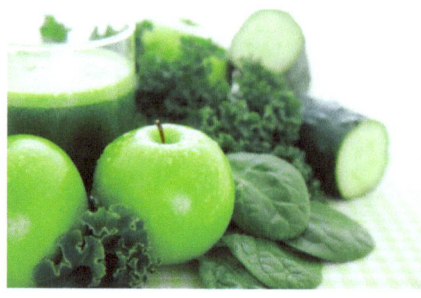

While most everybody loves fruit smoothies, many shy away from green smoothies. This is most likely due to a bad first experience with the green, leafy champion of smoothies. Let's face it blended greens can be less than palatable and downright nasty…IF not prepared properly. After all what good is a green smoothie if you can't get it past your lips and down the hatch? I guarantee after trying some of my favorite green smoothie recipes you'll soon change your tune; any bad experience you've had with the mean-green smoothie will long be forgotten.

Super green smoothies are indeed the champion of blended drinks, and rightfully so, due to the immense healing properties delivered by its rich chlorophyll content. The molecular structure of chlorophyll is almost identical to that of hemoglobin. Hemoglobin is the protein structure found in the blood. It carries oxygen from the lungs to the rest of the body, where it releases the oxygen to burn nutrients that provide energy for the process of metabolism. Hemoglobin makes up 96% +/- of the red blood cells content by weight.

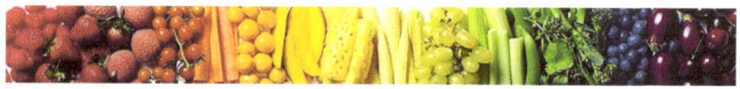

The main difference between hemoglobin and chlorophyll is that hemoglobin is built around iron (Fe) atom, where as chlorophyll is built around magnesium, (Mg).

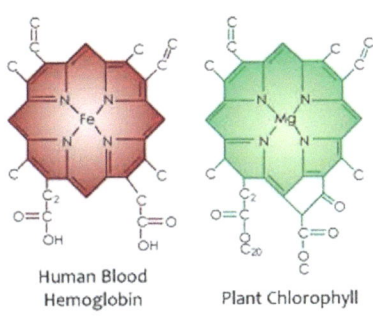

Human Blood Hemoglobin   Plant Chlorophyll

These similarities are impressive. Hemoglobin is composed of the four elements carbon, hydrogen, oxygen and nitrogen organized around iron. Chlorophyll is composed of the same elements, but are organized around magnesium.

Scientists have found chlorophyll to have anti-oxidant, anti-inflammatory and wound healing potential; its many benefits include:

1. The growth and repair of tissue.
2. Increased distribution of oxygen throughout the body.
3. Improving oxygen supply to red blood cells.
4. Deodorizing bad breath, urine, fecal waste and body odor.
5. Helping the body reduce toxins.

So, the next time you turn your nose up to green smoothies, consider the benefits. The good news is that green smoothies need not have that green grassy flavor. **Of course green smoothies are only as good as the blender that make**s them - as is true with all smoothies. When blending greens the last thing you want is a mouthful of chunky, stringy, fibrous goop.

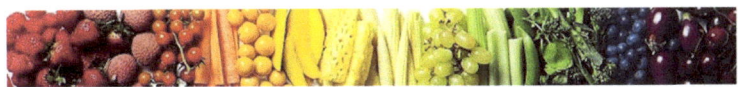

No worries, with the LifeEnergy Blender every recipe will deliver the richest, smoothest, creamiest green drink ever to pass your lips.

Here is a good formula to follow:

1 CUP Liquid Base	+	1 CUP Leafy Greens	+	2 CUPS Ripe Fruit
Pure Water		Kale		Apples
Coconut Water		Spinach		Avocado
Almond Milk		Spring Mix		Bananna
Coconut Milk		Dandelion		Berries
Green Tea		Swiss Chard		Kiwi
Peppermint Tea		Parsley		Lemon
Ginger Tea		Sprouts		Mango
				Peaches
				Pear
				Pineapple
				Plums

Yields approx 16 oz

Of course there are countless variations to the ingredients you may want to use, but by following this basic formula you are more likely to achieve the flavor and consistency desired.

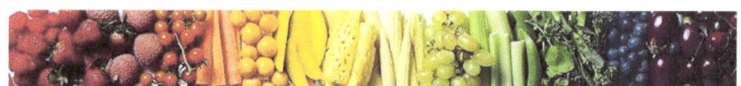

Every smoothie has a purpose. Some smoothies boost energy, other blends support healthy weight loss, still others provide an excellent way to recover from a workout. There are smoothies that assist in detoxing the body, and supplementing one's diet with the daily requirements of fruits and vegetables. But the main purpose of smoothies is to improve nutrition intake, and create greater health and wellness.

Regardless of why you choose to include smoothies in your diet, more importantly is that you make it a daily habit. The following table guides you through a typical week of smoothies. I prefer making my smoothies first thing in the morning - it's a great way to start the day!

DAY 1	DAY 2	DAY 3	DAY 4	DAY 5	DAY 6	DAY 7
2 C LIQUID BASE	1C LIQUID BASE	2C LIQUID BASE	1C LIQUID BASE	2C LIQUID BASE	2C LIQUID BASE	2C LIQUID BASE
3C LEAFY GREENS	2C LEAFY GREENS	1C LEAFY GREENS	2C LEAFY GREENS	1C LEAFY GREENS	1C LEAFY GREENS	3C LEAFY GREENS
1 BANANA	2 STALKS CELERY	1C KALE	1 AVOCADO	2C KALE	1C KALE	2 STALKS CELERY
2C FROZEN FRUIT	1C PINEAPPLE	1 BANANA	1C FROZEN FRUIT	1C PINEAPPLE	1 BANANA	1 AVOCADO
SUPER FOOD	1 ORANGE	1 APPLE	1 APPLE	1 ORANGE	1C FROZEN FRUIT	1 ORANGE
	1C ICE	1C ICE	SUPER FOOD	1C ICE	SUPER FOOD	1C ICE

Mix it up by substituting any of the recipes provided in the next chapter for any given day. As you explore the wonderful world of smoothies, you'll find many variations beyond the recipes provided. Have fun with it, and discover your own favorite blends. Remember, for an added boost, super-foods are a healthy addition to any smoothie.

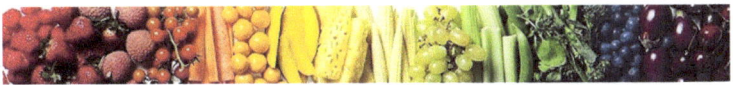

Chapter 5

Smoothies Galore
Best Recipes

So now that we have our basic formula, and have laid the foundation of knowledge, let's put all we have learned to the task of enjoying the many delicious recipes we can make with our LifeEnergy Blender. Keep in mind that any of the super-foods listed in Chapter 3: Healthy Additions may be considered in all of the following recipes.

Amazing Avocado

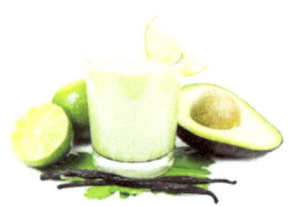

- 2 cups coconut milk
- 1 granny smith apple
- 2 cups fresh leafy greens
- 1 whole peeled avocado w/pit
- ½ lime unpeeled
- ½ tsp vanilla extract
- 1 bunch fresh mint

Makes approx. 3½ cups

Avocado puts the smooth in smoothie, it has a silky rich, creamy texture with so many amazing health benefits. Avocado pits increase the total antioxidant and phenolic content of this smoothie, while providing extra calcium, magnesium, phosphorus and potassium, and that's the truth! Now I dare you to try it - bet you can't sense the pit.

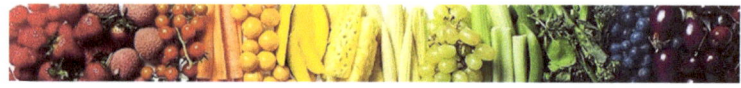

Granny's Green Green Tea

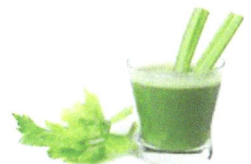

- 2 cups unsweetened green tea
- ½ lemon partially peeled
- 2 cups fresh leafy greens
- 2 cups fresh pineapple
- 1 stalk celery
- Dash of cayenne pepper

Makes approx. 3½ cups

Green tea helps improve brain function, fat metabolism and contains many bioactive compounds that can improve your health. Try it and see if it makes you smarter.

Mom's Minty Green

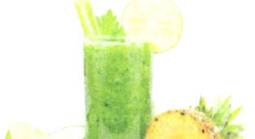

- 2 cups coconut water
- 1 green apple
- 1 bunch fresh mint
- ½ cup fresh parsley
- ½ cucumber
- ½ cup fresh pineapple
- ½ stalk celery
- ¼ lemon partially peeled
- ¼ orange partially peeled

Makes approx. 3½ cups

A refreshing high fiber, low calorie smoothie - day or night - to boost your energy. Full of anti-inflammatory enzymes, vitamin C, manganese, vitamin B1, and loads of antioxidants. When cutting pineapple be sure to include the core, and the crown of the pineapple, this is where most of the nutrients are.

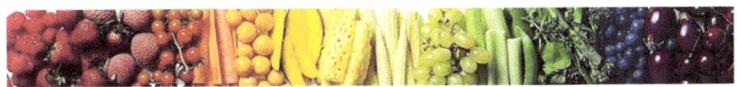

Royal Berry Blend

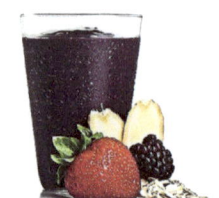

- 1 cup concord grape juice
- 1 cup almond milk
- 1 cup whole strawberries
- 1 cup leafy greens
- 1 cup blackberries
- 1 inch ginger
- 2 tbsp chia seeds
- ½ cup ice (optional)

Makes approx. 3½ cups

Loaded with antioxidants, research indicates blackberries may help reduce the risk of heart problems, periodontal disease and age-related decline in motor and cognitive function. Low in calories, high in fiber, and rich in nutrients - a great choice.

Kiwi Morning

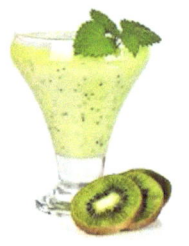

- 2 cups coconut water
- ½ cup green grapes
- 1 kiwi unpeeled
- ¼ cup broccoli stems & florets
- ½ lemon partially peeled
- 2 cups fresh leafy greens
- ½ green apple
- ½ cucumber
- 1 tbsp chia seeds

Makes approx. 3½ cups

Kiwi has more vitamin C than oranges, and about as much potassium as bananas. Kiwi is a natural blood thinner, and the skin is very high in omega-3 fatty acids as well as alpha-lipoid acids . These two acids are considered essential since they are not produced by the body, but must be acquired through our diet.

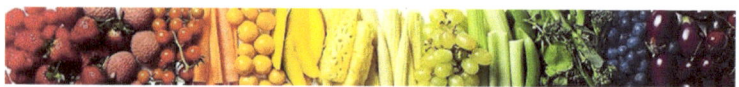

Red Banana Delight

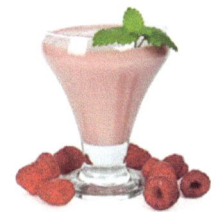

- 1 cup coconut water
- 1 cup coconut milk
- ¼ cup fresh beets
- 1 cup raspberries
- 1 cup ice (optional)
- 1 banana
- ½ cup whole strawberries

Makes approx. 3½ cups

Wonderfully delicious and creamy, this rich, red smoothie is full of nutrients, fiber, and antioxidants. Rich in beta-carotene, this combination plays a significant role against cancer, aging, inflammation, and neurodegenerative diseases.

Mad Vanilla Green

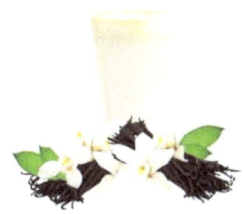

- 1 cup coconut milk
- 1 cup almond milk
- 2 tsp vanilla extract
- ½ cup vanilla yogurt
- ½ frozen banana
- 1 cup leafy greens
- 1 tsp maple syrup
- 1 tsp cinnamon

Makes approx. 3½ cups

This variation of the classic vanilla shake is a singular sensation. Add your favorite protein powder, and standby as your tastebuds go mad with delight - you'll think you're on Bourbon Island. This mellow-sweet, nutrient rich smoothie is perfect as a post-workout snack.

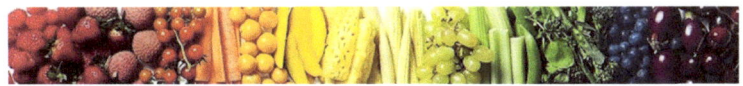

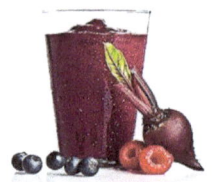

Uncle Vinny's Berry Beet-nick

- 1 cup cranberry juice
- 1 cup coconut milk
- 1 cup blueberries
- 1 cup fresh peeled beets
- ½ cup raspberries
- ½ cup yogurt
- 1 tsp maple syrup

Makes approx. 3½ cups

Loaded with vitamin A, B and C, this antioxidant, probiotic rich smoothie is one of a kind. Even the pickiest of eaters will give this smoothie a thumbs up. Beets are particularly beneficial to women, promoting new cell growth during pregnancy, and replenishing iron reserves. Beets are very medicinal, acting as a blood purifier and tonic for the liver. High in boron, beets are directly related to the production of sex hormones. Used as an aphrodisiac by ancient Romans, science now confirms that beet's are nature's Viagra.

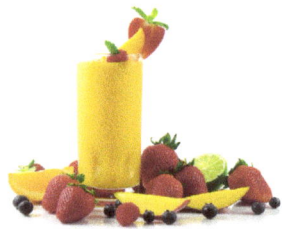

Mango Berry Cream

- 2 cups coconut milk
- 1 cup mango
- 1 cup leafy greens
- ¼ of a lime
- 1 orange with pith
- 1 cup plain yogurt
- ¼ cup whole strawberries
- 1 tbsp maple syrup

Makes approx. 3½ cups

A taste of the tropics that is sure to satisfy. Mango is considered "the king of fruits" due to its health promoting qualities. It is a pre-biotic dietary fiber, and a good source of potassium, vitamin A, B6, C, and E.

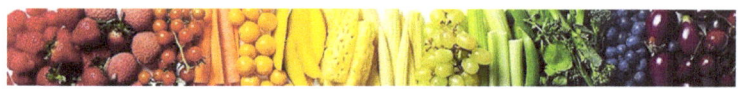

Power Punch

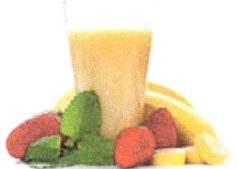

- 2 cups coconut water
- ½ cup whole strawberries
- 2 oranges peeled with pith
- 1 grapefruit peeled with pith
- 1 bunch fresh mint
- 1 cup kale
- 1 inch ginger

Makes approx. 3½ cups

Loaded with vitamin C, this stress busting, antioxidant rich smoothie can help boost your immunity. It packs a powerful punch in clearing the lungs and mucus membrane: 45 types of flavonoids provide antioxidant and anti-inflammatory power, while glucosinolates detox at a genetic level.

Verily Berrily

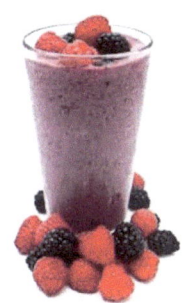

- 2 cups coconut water
- 1 cup blackberries
- 1 cup raspberries
- ½ cup yogurt
- 1 cup ice

Makes approx. 3½ cups

Just berries and cream - a fast, simple , refreshingly, juicy, delicious choice that is loaded with fiber, enhancing weight loss. One cup of berries daily is shown to improve cognition and motor skills.

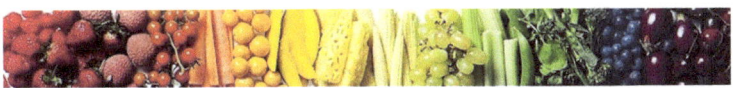

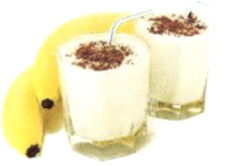

Hope's Banana-Rama Slammer

- 2 cups almond milk
- 2 bananas (fresh or frozen)
- 2 tbsp almonds
- 1 ½ tsp cinnamon
- 1 tsp pure maple syrup
- 4 oz frozen yogurt
- 1 tsp maca powder (optional)

Makes approx. 3½ cups

This smoothie is a big hit with children of all ages. Almonds may be substituted with ground nut butter of your choice. Maca is a great addition to this smoothie for its added nutrients and super-food power. Bananas are the only fruit that contains the amino acid tryptophan, plus vitamin B6, which helps the body produce serotonin - a natural antidepressant.

Shawn's Nutty-Buddy

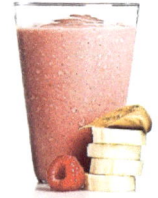

- 2 cups coconut water
- 1 cup raspberries
- 1 cup leafy greens
- 3 tbsp nut butter
- 1 banana
- 1 tbsp maple syrup
- 2 scoops hemp protein powder
- ½ cup ice

Makes approx. 3½ cups

For all you nut butter fans, this tasty, heart-healthy smoothie provides a generous dose of protein, antioxidants, minerals and vitamins. According to the Mayo Clinic nuts have several health benefits, including lowering cholesterol, regulate blood pressure, and reduce the risk of heart disease.

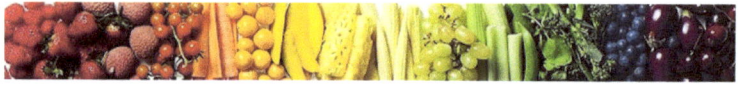

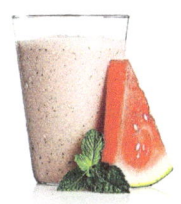

Minty Melon

- 2 cups almond milk
- 2 cups watermelon (with rind)
- 1 bunch fresh mint
- 1 cup leafy greens
- 1 cup blackberries
- 1 inch ginger
- 1 tbsp maple syrup

Makes approx. 3½ cups

Melons and blackberries are rich in fiber, and nutrients that may help control blood pressure, regulate heart beat, prevent kidney stones, bone-loss, and possibly prevent strokes, periodontal disease and age-related decline in motor and cognitive function. Low in calories, high in fiber and rich in nutrients - a great choice.

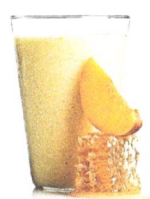

Peaches-n-Green

- 2 cups kefir
- 1 ½ cups fresh peaches
- 1 cup leafy greens
- ½ cup bee pollen
- 2 tsp honey
- 1 inch fresh turmeric
- ½ banana
- ½ cup ice

Makes approx. 3½ cups

This delightful smoothie has bioactive compounds with anti-inflammatory properties, high fiber, minerals and vitamin C. A truly holistic recipe.

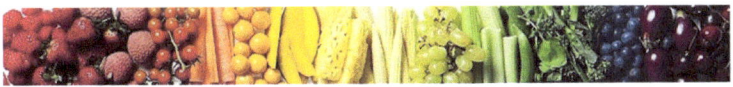

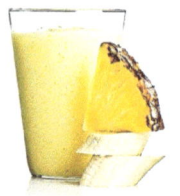

Banan-a-Colada

- 2 cups coconut milk
- ½ banana
- 1 cup leafy greens
- 1 cup fresh pineapple
- 1 cup fresh coconut
- 1 tsp vanilla extract
- 1 tsp maple syrup

Makes approx. 3½ cups

The sweet flavor of pineapple and coconut blends to create a soothing smoothie to be enjoyed anytime. Abundant in calcium, this smoothie helps maintain strong bones, and provides adequate levels of iron, potassium, vitamin A, B, C and E. Rich in lauric acid this smoothie is a power-house of healing energy with anti-viral, and anti-fungal properties.

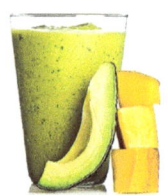

Basil Mango Mint

- 2 cups coconut milk
- 1 cup mango
- 1 cup leafy greens
- ½ avocado
- 1 bunch fresh mint
- ½ lime with pith
- 2 sprigs fresh basil leaves
- 1 tbsp maple syrup

Makes approx. 3½ cups

This delicious smoothie offers a healthy dose of essential fats that help protect against liver damage. This smoothie has it all. Load up on your fiber, protein, minerals, vitamins A, B, C, E, and K, while benefitting from its anti-inflammatory, anti-viral, and anti-fungal properties.

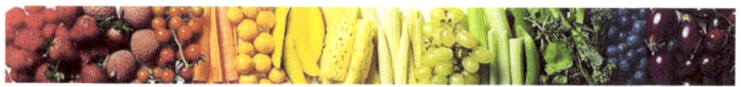

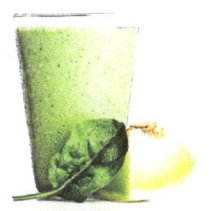

Honey I Dew

- 2 cups almond milk
- ⅓ cup yogurt
- 1 cup baby spinach
- 1 cup fresh honeydew melon
- ½ cup ice (optional)

Makes approx. 3½ cups

Simply good! Abundant in iron, fiber, vitamins B, C, K and essential nutrients for healthy skin and hair. Spinach is one of the best sources of dietary potassium, and magnesium, which is necessary for energy metabolism, maintaining muscle, nerve function, heart rhythm and a healthy immune system.

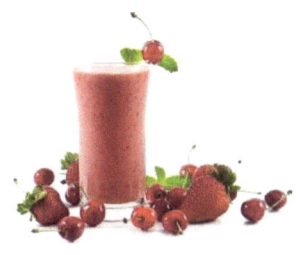

Go-go Berry

- 1 cup coconut water
- ½ cup pomegranate juice
- 1 cup leafy greens
- ½ cup goji berries
- 1 cup whole strawberries
- 1 cup pitted cherries
- 1 bunch of fresh mint
- 2 tbsp chia seeds

Makes approx. 3½ cups

A combination of essential fats, and goji to help control blood sugars and appetite. Goji is acclaimed as the most nutritionally dense food on Earth. It is both a fruit and an herb, with all essential amino acids, high beta-carotene, fiber, vitamin C, and twenty-one trace minerals. Chia provides sustainable energy - these seeds may be tiny, but they are packed with power to keep you going strong.

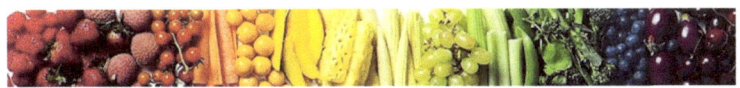

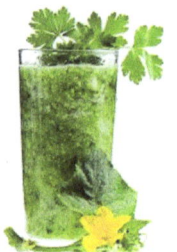

Rae's Green Power Machine

- 2 cups almond milk
- 1 cup each of kale
- 1 cup baby spinach
- 1 cup fresh pineapple
- 2 tbsp chia seeds
- 2 scoops protein powder

Makes approx. 3½ cups

Ultimate green power smoothie. Only for the serious minded, high achievers. This smoothie goes the distance, delivering high speed octane that just won't quit! A nutritional powerhouse that goes to bat against arthritis, asthma, autoimmune disorders, and cancer. This smoothie takes you the extra inning.

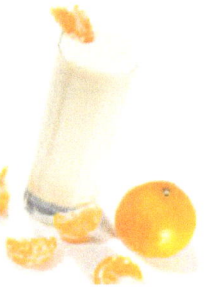

T-shirt Mike's Dreamsicle

- 1 cup coconut milk
- 1 cup almond milk
- 3 clementines with pith
- 2 oranges with pith
- 2 tbsp maca powder
- 2 scoops hemp protein powder
- ½ cup frozen vanilla yogurt
- ½ tsp vanilla extract

Makes approx. 3½ cups

A dreamy, delicious way to load up on vitamin C, reminiscent of hot summer days of childhood. A great cool down after shooting hoops. No foul will be called for leaning into this smoothie - it's all net - guaranteed!

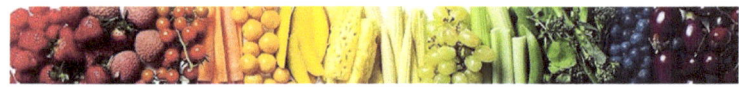

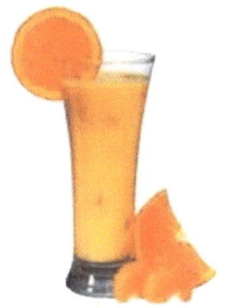

Own Ur Happy

- 2 cups coconut milk
- 1 cup papaya
- 1 cup orange with pith
- 1 cup yogurt
- 1 inch turmeric root
- 1 tbsp maple syrup
- ⅛ tsp rosewater
- 1 inch ginger (optional)
- ½ cup ice (optional)

Makes approx. 3½ cups

So good you're gonna want to share it. Papaya is rich in nutritional and medicinal properties. Mayans revered it as the "Tree of Life". Every part of the plant has medicinal properties, the leaves, seeds, and milk of the tree are used to cure intestinal problems, and kill intestinal worms and parasites. Now that's something to be happy about!

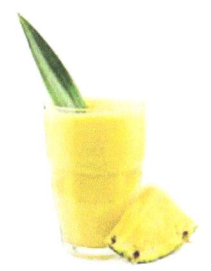

V's Cellular Defense

- 1 cup peppermint tea
- 1 cup green tea
- 1 cup pineapple
- 1 inch turmeric root
- 1 inch ginger root
- 1 lemon mostly peeled
- 2 sprigs fresh mint
- 2 sprigs fresh thyme
- 1 tbsp maple syrup

Makes approx. 3½ cups

Calculating the number of cells in our bodies is a monumental task, but caring for them need not be. Try this phenomenal smoothie, and leave the rest to nature.

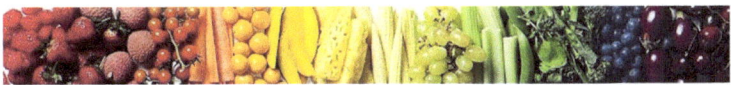

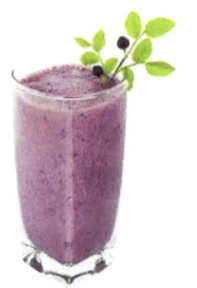

Bonnie's Blueberry Bliss

- 1 cup coconut water
- 2 cups blueberries
- ½ banana
- 1 cup yogurt
- 1 cup parsley, cilantro & mint
- 1 inch ginger
- 1 inch turmeric
- ½ lemon

Makes approx. 3½ cups

A truly blissful way to start your day. Blueberries offer tremendous benefits to the nervous system, and research suggests blueberries can improve memory, and strengthen and support every body system, making this smoothie an amazing choice.

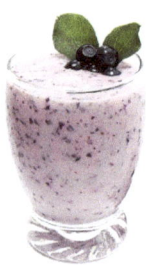

Just Bee Cause

- 2 cups coconut milk
- 1 cup yogurt
- 1 cup blueberries
- ½ cup bee pollen
- ⅛ tsp vanilla
- 2 tbsp chia seed
- ½ cup ice (optional)

Makes approx. 3½ cups

Another creamy smoothie packed with probiotics, antioxidants, and super nutrients that are sure to please the palate, and bring healing to the body.

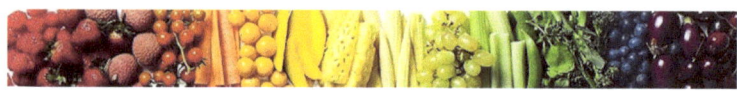

4 Baby-n-Me

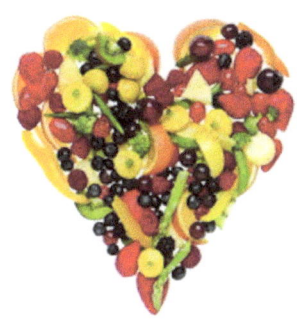

- 1 cup coconut water
- ½ avocado
- ½ banana
- ¼ cup mango
- ¼ cup papaya
- ¼ apple
- ½ peach
- 1 cup sunflower sprouts
  (after 12 mos. of age)
- 1 tsp fresh lemon juice
- 1 tsp maple syrup

Makes approx. 3½ cups

Smoothies are a delicious, and easy way to add nutrients to a child's diet. It's a delightful sight to watch little ones slurp away happily at theses nutritious, creamy blends.

Coconut water is a perfect addition to a child's diet, supplying essential vitamins, minerals and electrolytes. Coconut's antimicrobial properties are most useful as a preventive, and as a remedy for the tender digestive and urinary tract of your little one.

Creamy avocado, banana, papaya, mango, apple and peaches are excellent first foods to introduce to children, starting at 4 months of age.

Sprouts are very rich in chlorophyll, vitamin E, zinc, protein, and B vitamins, all of which support a strong immune system.

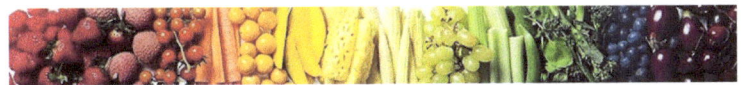

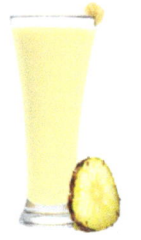

BJ's Grand Slam

- 2 cups coconut milk
- 1 cup kombucha
- 1 cup papaya
- 1 cup pineapple
- ½ cup mango
- ½ cup blueberries
- ½ cup raspberries
- 1 inch ginger
- ½ cup ice

Makes approx. 3½ cups

Wow! This creamy smoothie is packed with probiotics, antioxidants, and anti-inflammatory properties. This smoothie is a definite winner - giving you every advantage. A good match for any time of day. Guaranteed your gonna love it!

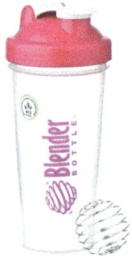

One 4 the Road

- 2 cups almond milk
- 1 cup cranberry juice
- 1 whole apple
- 2 bananas
- 2 tbsp protein powder
- 2 tbsp chia seeds
- ½ cup ice

Makes approx. 3½ cups

Out the door in less than 60 seconds! Take this delicious smoothie with you. Its packed with all the necessary nutrients to get you going, and keep you going down the road - come what may.

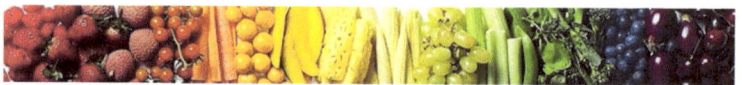

In Closing
Why Blend?

In answering the question *(why blend?)* we have established that using the LifeEnergy Blender has many benefits which include:

* An easy and convenient way to quickly boost your daily intake of vital nutrients

* Nutritious way to detox, drop extra pounds, stop disease and reverse aging

* Improve all body functions, increase energy, feel more alert, and be more active and productive

* Build strong cellular structures for healthy organs, glands, bones, and body systems,

* Improve eyesight, hair, skin, and nails

* Build a strong, lean, healthy body, reduce stress, improve fitness recovery, and promote healthy sleep

* Increases vitamin, enzyme, protein and mineral intake, and puts you on the fast-track to achieving optimum health

* A great way to get our children to drink their fruits and vegetables - and like it!

* Using the LifeEnergy Blender is also ideal for making healthy "baby foods"

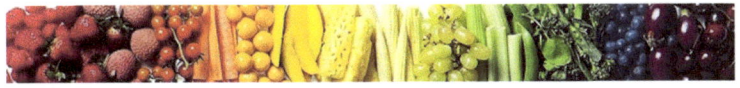

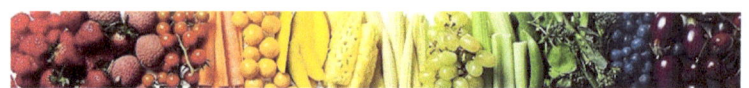

So the question is no longer

"to blend or not to blend"

but rather

...**are you ready to get started?**

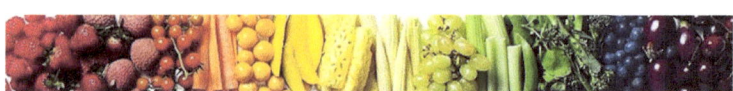

Invitation
For Your Name's Sake

Got a recipe you think would be enjoyed by others? Send it to us. Also send your name, and 3 of your favorite base ingredients (liquid, greens, fruit), and we will create a recipe that has your name sake, and we'll add it to the next edition of LifeEnergy Recipes.

Send to: LifeEnergy USA

                email@LifeEnergyUSA.com

We look forward to hearing from you!
Until then Happy Blending!

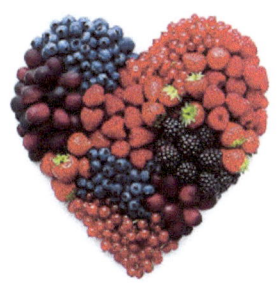

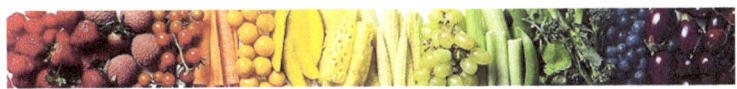

References

1. Clement, Charles R.; de Cristo-Araújo, Michelly; d'Eeckenbrugge, Geo Coppens; Alves Pereira, Alessandro; Picanço-Rodrigues, Doriane (6 January 2010). "Origin and Domestication of Native Amazonian Crops". Diversity 2 (1): 72–106. doi:10.3390/d2010072. Retrieved 9 November 2012.

2. Stegner, Mabel. 1940. "Let the Blender Do It for You!" New York Herald Tribune, This Week magazine. June 23. p. 14-15

3. Mischoulon D, Raab MF. The role of folate in depression and dementia. J Clin Psychiatry. 2007; 68[suppl 10]:28–33.

4. The Waring Corporation. 1940. Recipes to Make your Waring-Go-Round. New York, NY: The Waring Corporation. 48 p.

5. Fashner J, Ericson K, Werner S. Treatment of the common cold in children and adults. Am Fam Physician. 2012; 15; 86(2):153–9.

6. Slavin JL. Position of the American Dietetic Association: Health implications of dietary fiber. J Am Diet Assoc. 2008; 108:1716–1731.

7. Brown, Ellen (2005). The Complete Idiot's Guide to Smoothies.

8. Cosgrove MC, Franco OH, Granger SP, Murray PG, Mayes AE. Dietary nutrient intakes and skin-aging appearance among middle-aged American women. Am J Clin Nutr. 2007; 86:1225–1231.

9. Kohlenberg-Mueller K, Raschka L. Calcium balance in young adults on a vegan and lactovegetarian diet. J Bone Miner Metab. 2003; 21:28–33.

10. Haddy FJ, Vanhoutte PM, Feletou M. Role of potassium in regulating blood flow and blood pressure. Am J Physiol Regul Integr Comp Physiol. 2006; 290:R546-R552.